ICS 03.180

SCM

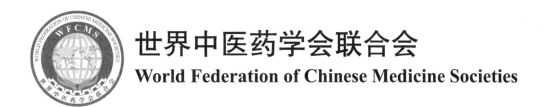

世界中医药学会联合会

World Federation of Chinese Medicine Societies

SCM 0012-2014

国际中医医师测试与评审规范

Test and Assessment Procedures of International Chinese Medicine Doctors

2014-10-02 发布实施

中国中医药出版社

图书在版编目（CIP）数据

国际中医医师测试与评审规范/世界中医药学会联
合会著 . —北京：中国中医药出版社，2016.10
　ISBN 978-7-5132-3425-2

　Ⅰ.①国… Ⅱ.①世… Ⅲ.①中医师—测试—规范—
世界 ②中医师—评定—规范—世界 Ⅳ.①R2-65

中国版本图书馆 CIP 数据核字（2016）第 104229 号

中国中医药出版社出版
北京市朝阳区北三环东路 28 号易亨大厦 16 层
邮政编码　100013
传真　010 64405750
三河市潮河印业有限公司印刷
各地新华书店经销

*

开本 880×1230　1/16　印张 3　字数 83 千字
2016 年 10 月第 1 版　2016 年 10 月第 1 次印刷
书　号　ISBN 978-7-5132-3425-2

*

定价　38.00 元
网址　www.cptcm.com

目　　次

前　言

本标准主要起草单位：世界中医药学会联合会考试与测评委员会、世界中医药学会联合会资格考试部、北京中医药大学。

本标准主要起草人：郑跃先、高思华、高文柱、徐金香、李振吉、徐春波、翟双庆、张立平、唐民科、顾晓静、包文虎。

本标准参与起草人：

中国：姜再增、陈立新、谷晓红、丁霞、吴宇峰、秦树坤、肖俊平、赵百孝、闫晓天、杨抒宁、张华祚、孙奇、于树森、喻文迪。

新加坡：赵英杰。

巴西：史宏、马佩玲。

墨西哥：宋钦福、李美虹。

美国：金鸣。

匈牙利：于福年、夏林军。

加拿大：吴滨江。

日本：陈坚鹰。

瑞士：李一鸣。

意大利：何嘉琅。

本标准的起草，遵守了世界中医药学会联合会发布的 SCM 0001-2009《标准制定和发布工作规范》所规定的程序。

本标准在 2014 年 10 月 2 日俄罗斯召开的世界中医药学会联合会第三届第六次理事会上审议通过。

本标准由世界中医药学会联合会发布，版权归世界中医药学会联合会所有。

引　言

构建国际中医药人才标准体系，是国际中医药人才战略的重要组成部分。建立国际中医药人才测评标准，通过统一评价要素与指标，统一测评内容与方法，对各级各类中医药人才的知识结构和临床能力进行评价，是不断提高国际中医药人才整体素质、加快国际中医药人才战略实施进程的重要落脚点与支撑。

为促进国际中医药专业技术职称测评走上科学化、标准化轨道，在充分调研的基础上，依据国际标准制定的规定程序，组织起草了《国际中医医师测试与评审规范》（以下简称《测评规范》）。

本标准的制定，参考了美国、日本、英国等国家的医师管理相关法规、中国《执业医师法》、世界中医药学会联合会颁布的相关标准等文件，从规范国际中医医师测评的视角，对测评操作提出了相关要求。

本标准在各级中医医师理论知识结构与临床技术能力要求方面，注意了与 SCM 0003-2009《世界中医学本科（CMD 前）教育标准》附录 A，与《中医学本科（CMD 前）教育专业知识与技能基本要求》和 SCM 0010-2012《世界中医学专业核心课程》等相关标准的内容相衔接。

本标准以《国际中医医师专业技术职称分级标准》为依据，将中医医师分为助理医师、执业医师、专科医师、高级专科医师、主任医师五个级别。从中医医师成长规律出发，明确了助理医师、执业医师、专科医师三个层次，以纸笔作答、临床技术操作为主要方式，重点对考试者的"知识要素""能力要素"进行测评。高级专科医师及以上职称，通过论文评议、有效病案审核与论文答辩，对参评者的临床、科研、带教、创新意识等能力进行综合评价。

本标准旨在建立适用于世界大部分国家或地区的中医医师测评内容与方法、程序，为各国中医医师能力评估、各中医院校年度考试、教师水平评价等相关测评提供参考。各国可在本国（地区）相关法律法规框架下，合理参照本操作规范，建立适宜本国（地区）中医医师能力测评的管理办法，不断提高中医医师管理水平，保证中医医疗服务质量与安全，为保障全球人民的健康做出更大的贡献。

国际中医医师测试与评审规范

1 范围

本标准规定了针对中医医师开展测试与评审的基本内容、方法和程序。

本标准适用于从事或即将从事中医临床的各级、各专业中医医师中医理论水平与临床技术能力的水平认证。

2 规范性引用文件

下列文件对本文件的应用是必不可少的。凡是注日期的引用文件，仅注日期的版本适用于本文件。凡是不注日期的引用文件，其最新版本（包括所有的修改单）适用于本文件。

SCM 0003 世界中医学本科（CMD 前）教育标准

SCM 0008 国际中医医师专业技术职称分级标准

SCM 0010 世界中医学专业核心课程

3 术语和定义

下列术语和定义适用于本文件。

3.1 测试

通过笔试（纸笔作答）、临床技术操作的方式，对应试者中医理论水平和临床技能进行水平测试的过程。

3.2 评审

通过同行专家对参评者论文进行评议、对有效病案进行审核和论文答辩，对其中医理论、临床、科研、带教等水平进行评审的过程。

3.3 专业培训

以各种方式学习中医药理论与临床技能的过程。

3.4 临床实践

以中医药理论为指导，运用中医、针灸、推拿等专业知识从事中医临床的过程。

3.5 书面辨证论治

考生针对以书面形式提供的病例数据，依据中医理论进行辨证思维，做出病名与证型诊断，提出治法、方药（针灸、推拿选穴，操作方法）的过程。

4 相关方职责

4.1 测评机构

4.1.1 开展中医医师测评活动的机构应为中医药医疗、教育机构，中医药学会等社团，并具备以下基本条件：

（1）符合所在国家或地区规定的相关要求；

（2）有具备相应资质的命题、测试、评审专家与符合资质要求的执考人员；

（3）有开展相应测评所需的场地、设备、设施。

4.1.2 测评机构应成立由中医药各专业专家组成的测评委员会，并明确职责、工作程序等要求，并建立覆盖测评全程的管理规则，确保测评质量。

4.2 测评组织方

测评组织方应依据报名条件，完成考生资质初审与推荐，开展考生培训。

4.3 测评实施方

测评实施方对参加测评人员的资质进行复核，依据相关规则实施测评。

4.4 测评对象

4.4.1 中医医师测评的对象应为正在从事或经过系统学习，即将从事中医临床工作的人员。

4.4.2 参加测评者的学习和从业经历等，均应符合相应级别中医医师测评的资质要求。

5 测评分类

5.1 测试

5.1.1 测试以验证考生是否具备中医医师必须掌握的基本知识和技能为目的。

5.1.2 以笔试和临床技术操作为主要测试方法。

5.1.3 通过测试，可获得中医助理医师、执业医师或专科医师证书。

5.2 评审

5.2.1 应主要考核参评者专业理论与医疗、科研、带教等综合能力与水平。

5.2.2 以同行专家论文评议、病案审核、论文答辩为评审方式。

5.2.3 通过评审，临床系列可获得高级专科医师或主任医师职称。

6 测评方法

6.1 笔试

6.1.1 应用范围和形式

6.1.1.1 旨在考核中医基本医学理论、中医临床医学知识的掌握与应用能力。

6.1.1.2 主要采用选择题和书面辨证论治试题进行测试。

6.1.2 笔试科目

6.1.2.1 中医专业

测试中医基础理论、中医诊断学、中药学、方剂学、中医内科学、中医外科学、中医妇科学、中医儿科学相关知识和常见病、多发病的书面辨证论治。

6.1.2.1.1 中医专业（针灸方向）

测试中医基础学、正常人体解剖学、经络腧穴学、临床针灸学相关知识和常见病、多发病书面辨证论治。

6.1.2.1.2 中医专业（推拿方向）

测试中医基础学、正常人体解剖学、经络腧穴学、中医推拿学相关知识和常见病、多发病书面辨证论治。

6.1.2.1.3 中医专业（美容方向）

测试中医学基础、中药学与方剂学、中医美容基础知识、中医美容临床技术和常见损美性病证书面辨证论治。

6.1.2.1.4 中医专业（骨伤方向）

测试中医学基础、正常人体解剖学、经络腧穴学与推拿学、中医骨伤学相关知识和常见病、多发病书面辨证论治。

6.2 临床技术操作

6.2.1 旨在考核中医临床基本技能、解决临床实际问题的水平与能力。

6.2.2 主要对常规消毒、腧穴定位、常用毫针刺法、灸法、推拿、拔罐、正骨、理筋手法、小夹板固定等临床技术操作能力进行考核。

6.3 评审

6.3.1 采用同行评议方式。

6.3.2 重点对中医理论水平，临床、科研、带教以及中医经典理论掌握与应用能力做出评价。

6.4 论文答辩

6.4.1 论文答辩，是在论文评议的基础上，通过现场回答专家提出的问题，对参评人临床思维能力、科研素养、文献引述等方面进行综合评价。

6.4.2 通过针对论文表述的薄弱环节、相关学术论点、新理论、新疗法，以及论文涉及的相关诊断标准、疗效标准、相关数据等问题的答辩，重点考核临床思辨能力与中医科研素养。

7 测试工作流程

7.1 确定测试大纲

7.1.1 测评实施方应采用适当的方式公布测试大纲，以方便申请者在测试前获得。

7.1.2 测试大纲应明确规定测试的具体范围。

7.2 制定测试实施方案

明确测试题型、方式、分数、及格标准等相关内容。

7.3 遴选命题专家

7.3.1 命题专家应具有规定学历，原则上具有中医副主任医师及以上技术职称。

7.3.2 熟悉本专业理论与临床技能，了解本学科进展。

7.3.3 熟悉命审题技术规则。

7.4 明确命题任务

7.4.1 制定命题方案，明确题量、题型、认知层次、预计难度等相关参数。

7.4.2 确保测试范围合理覆盖了主要知识点。

7.5 命题基本规则

7.5.1 命题范围不得超出测试大纲。

7.5.2 试题考查的内容应全面覆盖主要知识点。

7.5.3 不应出偏题、怪题、冷僻题，并回避学术上有争议的内容。

7.5.4 试题内容应科学严谨。名词术语应准确，计量单位应规范。

7.5.5 一道试题应提出一个单一问题。

7.5.6 应避免易引起种族、宗教、残疾、性别歧视等误解的表述。

7.5.7 试题中的数字应统一用阿拉伯数字。

7.5.8 题干中的否定词应用黑体字加粗。

7.5.9 试题预计难度应分为难、较难、中，较易、易五个级别。

7.6 命题主要流程与要求

7.6.1 命题人应依据《命题方案》规定的参数做出命题计划，填写《命题细目表》。

7.6.2 确认《命题细目表》合理覆盖了主要知识点、各项参数逻辑关系正确后方可开始命题。

7.6.3 规范填写命题卡，不得遗漏任何项目。

7.6.4 准确标注试题标准答案出处（教材名称、版本、页码）。

7.6.5 准确提炼试题关键词。

7.6.6 自审"试题关键词"，确认无重复试题并分布合理。

7.6.7 自审全部命题，确认无错题、错字，并符合《命题方案》规定的参数后，提交试题复审。

7.7 题型结构

7.7.1 选择题

7.7.1.1 A_1型题

每道试题由 1 个题干和 5 个供选择的备选答案组成。题干以叙述式单句出现，备选答案中只有 1 个是最佳选择，称为正确答案。其余 4 个均为干扰答案。干扰答案可完全不正确或部分正确。

7.7.1.2 A_2型题

以一个简要的病例或两个以上相关因素作为题干，后面是与题干有关的 5 个备选答案。症状、舌质舌苔、脉象必须齐全。若病情与性别、年龄无关者，可略写性别、年龄。答题时，要求从中选择一项作为正确答案。

7.7.1.3 B₁型题

试题由若干个备选答案与两个或两个以上题干组成，备选答案在前，题干在后。答题时，要求为每个题干选择一项作为正确答案。每个备选答案可以选用一次或一次以上，也可以一次也不选用。

7.7.1.4 题干表述

题干表述应符合以下主要规则：

a）题干结尾均不加标点符号；

b）否定式提问试题比例不宜过大；

c）题干中不宜出现双重否定表达方式；

d）B₁型试题采用两个或两个以上题干共享5个备选答案，两个或两个以上题干表达形式要一致，内容应在同一范畴。

7.7.1.5 备选答案

备选答案设置应符合以下基本原则：

a）5个备选答案的内容应为同一范畴；

b）备选答案之间不得相互包容与提示；

c）如是数字，应按从小到大或从大到小顺序排列；

d）干扰答案应具有一定程度的迷惑性与干扰性。

7.7.1.6 正确答案

正确答案设置应符合以下基本原则：

a）以考试指定教材（指南）为依据；

b）准确标明正确答案的教材（指南）版本与具体页码。

7.7.2 技术操作试题

7.7.2.1 应重点考查相关专业的基本实际操作技能。

7.7.2.2 答案准确，评分标准公正合理。

7.7.3 书面辨证论治试题

7.7.3.1 书面辨证论治试题应准确提供以下信息：

a）患者姓名、性别、年龄、民族、婚况、出生地、职业、发病节气、病史陈述者；

b）主诉：应明确促使患者就诊的主要症状（或体征）及持续时间；

c）现病史：内容包括发病情况、主要症状、发展变化情况、诊疗经过等内容；

d）既往史：提供患者既往健康状况、疾病史、过敏史；

e）与中医辨证相关的个人史、婚育史、月经史、家族史。

7.7.3.2 书面辨证论治试题测试内容有：

a）诊断：做出中医病证诊断和证候诊断；

b）治法：针对病证诊断提出中医（针灸、推拿、骨伤、美容等）治疗方法；

c）处方：提出拟选用的方剂，针灸主、配穴，推拿部位、手法，正骨理筋手法，美容技术等；

d）药物组成依据病情对所选方剂中的药物（腧穴）进行合理加减、配伍；

e）方剂药物应标注剂量，注明剂数与煎服法，针灸处方应标明针刺手法等相关内容；

f）医嘱：主要提出相关调护要求。

7.8 审题规则

7.8.1 履行自审、复审、审定程序，确保试题质量。

7.8.2 主要审核内容应包括：

a）测试内容是否超出考试大纲；

b）题型结构是否正确；

c）题干所问是否清晰明了；

d）备选答案是否在同一范畴；

e）核准正确答案出处；

f）确认干扰选项均不是最佳的正确答案；

g）试题主题词提炼是否正确；

h）是否存在错字、别字。

7.9 题库建设

7.9.1 应设专人负责题库管理。

7.9.2 以考试科目名称为标识入库试题，每题设有唯一编号。

7.9.3 题库总量应根据测试需求确定。

7.9.4 各科目试题总量，应不少于入卷试题的 5 倍。

7.9.5 应根据大纲变化和考试目标的变更，定期更新与补充试题。

7.9.6 严格执行相关保密规定，确保题库安全。

7.10 组卷

7.10.1 应根据考生层次、考试目的制定《组卷方案》。

7.10.2 《组卷方案》应明确规定题型比例、预计难度、认知层次等各项参数要求。

7.10.3 入卷试题应合理覆盖主要知识点。

7.10.4 依据考试规则，每次考试原则上要组合 A 与 B 两套试卷。

7.10.5 确保 A 与 B 两套试卷基本等值。

7.11 审卷

7.11.1 组卷完成后，依据"7.8.审题规则"，至少应有 2 人对试卷中的每道试题进行复审。发现问题，交组卷人修改完善。

7.11.2 资深专家完成试卷复审。

7.11.3 命题部门负责人完成试题审定。

7.12 试卷入库

7.12.1 按考试科目分别入库。

7.12.2 每卷有唯一编码。

7.12.3 按专业、组卷时间登记。

7.13 试卷启用

7.13.1 履行三级审卷程序。

7.13.2 对启用时间、应用国家（地区）进行准确登记。

7.14 试卷印制与保管

7.14.1 至少 2 人共同完成首份试卷印制与分拣、装订。

7.14.2 对试卷所载题量、题号顺序、页码接续等是否正确进行审核。

7.14.3 考务人员履行审读职责。确认无误后，完成试卷印制。

7.14.4 至少 2 人对试题序号接续、各页面试题完整性、试卷页码接续等内容再次复核。

7.14.5 核准试卷印制数量，放保密柜封存。

7.15 统计分析

7.15.1 测试后应对试题的区分度进行统计分析。

7.15.2 创造条件对试题的实测难度进行标注。

7.15.3　如具备条件，应开展试题信度、效度分析，试题与试卷的等值分析。

7.16　考务管理

7.16.1　考试报名

7.16.1.1　报名信息应提前公布，并提供考试相关咨询。

7.16.1.2　报考人员应在规定的时间内提交报名表及相关证明材料。

7.16.1.3　测评实施方对报考人员个人信息及资质进行审核后发放准考证。

7.16.2　执考人员

7.16.2.1　包括主考1人，监考1人。有临床技术操作考试的专业，执考人员中至少应有1名相应专业专家。

7.16.2.2　可根据需要设置翻译人员。

7.16.3　主考条件

7.16.3.1　具有中医药专业正高级职称，熟悉考试管理规则。

7.16.3.2　能够廉洁自律，公正执考，并能自觉遵守保密纪律。

7.16.3.3　有较强的考试管理与协调能力。

7.16.4　主考职责

7.16.4.1　依据考试管理相关规定负责考试实施。

7.16.4.2　妥善处理考试期间发生的突发事件。

7.16.5　监考条件

7.16.5.1　具有中医药专业中级及以上技术职称，熟悉考试管理规则。

7.16.5.2　能廉洁自律，公正执考，并能自觉遵守保密纪律。

7.16.6　监考职责

7.16.6.1　协助主考做好考场相关管理工作。

7.16.6.2　完成主考交给的各项工作任务。

7.16.6.3　负责答题卡回收、密封，安排操作考试等工作事项。

7.16.7　翻译条件

7.16.7.1　应精通考试所用语种，至少具有3年以上专业翻译工作经历。

7.16.7.2　熟悉中医药专业知识。

7.16.8　翻译职责

7.16.8.1　承担考场翻译任务，准确翻译提问与回答内容，不得违背原意。

7.16.8.2　遵守考试管理规则，不擅自对考生进行提示。

7.16.9　考试规则

7.16.9.1　测评机构应制定考场规则，规范考生行为，并明确相应处罚措施。

7.16.9.2　测评机构应制定执考守则，规范执考行为，保证考试公平、公正。

7.16.10　考场布置

7.16.10.1　考场应选择在交通方便、周边安静的区域。

7.16.10.2　考试排程应张贴在考场显著位置。

7.16.10.3　考生单排单桌，前后左右间距应不少于80厘米。

7.16.10.4　按顺序在考桌左上角张贴考号。

7.16.11　考前准备

7.16.11.1　执考人员应依据考试日程表逐一核对试卷信息和相关考试用品。

7.16.11.2　执考人员应按照考场布置的要求对考场进行仔细检查。

7.16.12　考试流程

7.16.12.1 笔试

7.16.12.1.1 开考前由主考介绍执考团队成员、考场规则、考试相关信息和注意事项。

7.16.12.1.2 启封试卷：执考人员向考生展示试卷密封完好无损后方可启封试卷袋。

7.16.12.1.3 发放试卷：试卷、答题卡、草稿纸应由执考人员发放，不得由考生互传。

7.16.12.1.4 主考宣布考试开始，考生方可开始答题。

7.16.12.1.5 核对信息：监考人员对考生信息、准考证照片、有效证件照片进行审验。发现问题，及时向主考报告。

7.16.12.1.6 结束提示：考试结束前20分钟，执考人员应提示考生注意时间。

7.16.12.1.7 考试结束：考试结束信号发出后，考生应停止答卷，将试卷与答题卡放在桌面上，退离考场。

7.16.12.1.8 密封试卷：执考人员按号码顺序收集整理答题卡，连同考场记录一同装入答题卡专用袋密封。

7.16.12.1.9 至少2人签署姓名与时间。

7.16.12.2 临床操作

7.16.12.2.1 抽题备考：考生应提前5分钟在准备区随机抽取试题备考。

7.16.12.2.2 技术操作：考生逐一进入考场，叙述并演示技术操作内容。

7.16.12.2.3 评分：至少有2名执考人员依据标准答案各自评分，计算平均值为考生成绩。

7.16.12.2.4 密封试卷：考试结束，执考人员应将考生成绩单和试卷装袋密封并签字。

7.16.13 执考报告

执考报告应覆盖以下内容：

a) 考试专业、期次、考生人数（初考、补考）、考试国家、考场所在城市、考试组织方（团体或个人）；

b) 考生资质：国籍、学历、职业、年龄相关情况；

c) 该考点既往组织考试情况：考试专业、级别、期次、各年度考生人数；高级职称评审人数与评审时间；

d) 存在的主要问题：主要涉及考务管理、试卷试题质量等方面；考试组织方主要意见和建议；

e) 考试拓展相关情况；

f) 执考团队体会与建议。

7.17 阅卷

7.17.1 考务管理人员与阅卷人填写《试卷及答题卡交接清单》。

7.17.2 阅卷人应具有中医药专业技术职称。

7.17.3 应在指定场所集体阅卷，试卷及答题卡不得带出阅卷场所。

7.17.4 依据试题管理处提供的标准答案，用红笔评阅试卷。

7.17.5 同一份试卷至少由2人评阅。完成阅卷后在指定位置签名。

7.17.6 阅卷复核人认真复核成绩。如遇错评，纠正后签署签名。如有争议，由考试部门领导裁定。

7.17.7 原则上考试完成后3周内完成阅卷与成绩统计。

7.17.8 成绩登录后，任何人不得擅自更改考生成绩。

7.18 档案管理

7.18.1 应制定档案管理制度。

7.18.2 档案管理制度应明确考生信息、答题卡、成绩单等数据和文件资料的存贮、使用和管理。

8 评审工作流程

8.1 申请程序

8.1.1 评审机构应明确参评者学历、从业年限等资质要求。

8.1.2 申请人如实填写申请表各项内容，并对本人在从业期间有否违背法律法规等不良记录做如实申明。

8.1.3 评审组织方应依据评审机构对参评者学历、从业年限等资质要求，对申请人数据进行初审。

8.1.4 对符合资质要求者，由所在单位（社团、院校等）或2名具有中医药高级职称者出具推荐意见。

8.2 提交评审资料

8.2.1 公开发表的中医学术论文2篇，每篇不少于3000字。

8.2.2 覆盖5个及以上不同病证的有效病案至少10个。

8.2.3 以英文以外其他小语种撰写论文者，需提供中文与英文摘要。

8.3 资质审查

测评机构应对申报材料进行审查，确认申请人是否具备参评资格。

8.4 同行评审

8.4.1 应根据论文和病案内容，选择2名及以上同专业专家进行评审。

8.4.2 评审专家原则上应具有主任医师、教授、研究员职称。

8.4.3 论文和病案应在论文答辩前2个月送审。

8.4.4 论文评议的主要内容应包括：

a）中医临床思维的连贯性；

b）中医理论应用的正确性；

c）中医临床研究的科学性；

d）文献引述的准确性；

e）相关资料的真实性；

f）临床治疗的有效性；

g）临床研究的创新性；

h）相关分析的逻辑性；

i）论文结论的严谨性；

j）指导临床的可用性。

8.4.5 病案评审的主要内容应包括：

a）病例的真实性；病案描述的逻辑性、准确性；

b）中医病证、证型诊断的正确性；

c）治法、方药（主穴、配穴、推拿、正骨等手法）的合理性；

d）疗程的可信性；

e）其他与病案相关的问题。

8.4.6 评审意见

8.4.6.1 测评机构应根据同行评议情况，做出以下评审意见：

a）达到相应水平，同意参加答辩；

b）建议对论文、病案进行完善，暂不同意参加答辩。

8.4.6.2 测评机构应及时向参评者回馈评审结论。

8.5 实施论文答辩

8.5.1 答辩委员会应由 5~7 名具有主任医（药）师、教授、研究员职称的相关专业专家组成。

8.5.2 参评人报告论文摘要 15 分钟，专家提问及答辩共计 25 分钟。

8.5.3 如需用中文以外的语种答辩，可合理增加答辩时间 10~15 分钟，翻译人员应做出准确翻译的承诺。

8.5.4 答辩委员会专家分别独立评分。

8.5.5 统计评分情况后，答辩委员会讨论并做出如下结论：

a）通过答辩；

b）论文需修改后再行审议；

c）未通过答辩。

8.5.6 报国际中医药专业技术职称评审委员会审批。

8.6 评审结果

8.6.1 考试和评审结果报测评委员会审定。

8.6.2 及时、准确公布评审结果。

9 证书管理

9.1 依据测评委员会审定结果为通过测评者制作证书。

9.2 2 个月内完成证书公证。

9.3 如遇有参评人资质虚假、不良记录没有如实申明等情形，评审机构可撤销已发放的评审证书，并通报考试组织方。

附录 A

（资料性）
题型示例

A.1 选择题示例

A.1.1 A₁型题示例

其性重浊的邪气是 （叙述式）

A. 风

B. 暑

C. 湿

D. 燥

E. 寒

答案：C

A.1.2 A₂型题示例

A.1.2.1 示例一

患者健忘失眠，眩晕耳鸣，五心烦热，胁痛腰酸，口干咽燥，舌红少津，脉细数。其证候是

A. 肾阴虚

B. 心阴虚

C. 肝肾阴虚

D. 肝血虚

E. 肺肾阴虚

答案：C

A.1.2.2 示例二

患者，女，28 岁，已婚。妊娠后小腹胁肋胀痛，急躁易怒，舌苔薄黄，脉弦滑。治疗应首选的方剂是

A. 逍遥散

B. 小柴胡汤

C. 大柴胡汤

D. 胶艾汤

E. 当归芍药散

答案：A

A.1.3 B₁型题示例

A. 肝

B. 心

C. 脾

D. 肺

E. 肾

濡养筋脉，使人体耐受疲劳的脏器是 答案：A

与四肢的营养状况关系最密切的脏器是 答案：C

A.2 书面辨证论治试题示例

患者姓名	＊＊＊	性别	男	年龄	6 岁	婚否	未婚	职业	银行职员
居住地	中国·北京市西城区					初诊日期	2007 年 1 月 3 日		

问诊：

主诉：恶寒发热 1 天。

现病史：昨日下午开始感到身体不适，怕冷发热，逐渐加重。当前恶寒发热，恶寒重，发热轻，无汗，头痛，鼻塞，时流清涕，喷嚏频作，咽痒，咳痰清稀色白。

既往史：健康。

望诊：舌苔薄白而润。

闻诊：语声重浊。

切诊：脉浮紧。

参考答案

诊断：病名诊断：感冒。

证型诊断：风寒（风寒束表）。

治法：辛温解表，宣肺散寒。

处方：荆防败毒散加减。

荆芥 6g　防风 6g　羌活 6g　独活 6g

柴胡 6g　川芎 6g　前胡 6g　茯苓 6g

枳壳 6g　桔梗 6g　甘草 3g

3 剂。每日 1 剂，水煎去滓取汁，早晚分服。

医嘱：避风寒，多休息，慎饮食，忌生冷油腻。

医师签名：＊＊＊

处方时间：2007 年 1 月 3 日

A.3 临床操作试题示例

A.3.1 示例一

请按要求确定地仓（ST 4）穴在人体的具体位置，并简述取穴依据或要领。

答案：在面部，口角外侧，上直瞳孔。

A.3.2 示例二

夹持进针法。

答案：或称骈指进针法，即用左手拇、食二指持捏消毒干棉球，夹住针身下端，将针尖固定在所刺腧穴的皮肤表面位置，右手捻动针柄，将针刺入腧穴。此法适用于长针的进针。

附录 B

（资料性）
国际中医医师级别设置与报名条件

B.1 级别设置

国际中医医师专业技术职称分为以下 5 个级别：

（1）助理医师

（2）执业医师

（3）专科医师

（4）高级专科医师

（5）主任医师

B.2 报名条件

B.2.1 助理医师

参加助理医师测试的人员应至少符合以下要求中的 1 项：

（1）取得中医实习医师职称后，临床实践 3 年以上。

（2）中医学中专学历（学制 3 年），中医临床实践 3 年以上。

（3）中医学大专学历（学制 3 年），中医临床实践 1 年以上。

（4）参加中医药学专业培训累计满 1500 学时，中医临床实践 1 年以上。

（5）家传、师承或自学中医，从事中医临床工作 5 年以上，经中医药学术团体或医疗机构推荐。

B.2.2 执业医师

参加执业医师测试的人员应至少符合以下要求中的 1 项：

（1）取得中医助理医师职称后，临床实践 3 年以上。

（2）取得中医硕士学位。

（3）中医学本科学历，临床实践 1 年以上。

（4）中医学大专学历，临床实践 3 年以上。

（5）中医学中专学历，临床实践 5 年以上。

（6）非医学类本科及以上学历，参加中医药学专业培训累计满 2500 学时（理论学习时间不少于 1500 学时），临床实践 1 年以上。

（7）以家传、师承、自学方式学习中医者，以中医为职业，临床实践 12 年以上，经中医药专业学术团体或医疗机构推荐。

B.2.3 专科医师

参加专科医师测试的人员应至少符合以下要求中的 1 项：

（1）取得中医执业医师职称后，临床实践 5 年以上。

（2）取得中医博士学位者。

（3）取得中医硕士学位后，临床实践 2 年以上。

（4）中医本科学历，临床实践 6 年以上。

（5）中医大专学历，临床实践 9 年以上。

（6）中医中专学历，临床实践 11 年以上。

（7）非医学类本科及以上学历，参加中医药学专业培训累计满 2500 学时（理论学习时间不少于

1500 学时），中医临床实践 6 年以上。

（8）家传、师承或自学中医，以中医为职业，从医满 17 年；或从医满 12 年，参加中医药学专业培训累计满 3000 学时（理论学习时间不少于 2000 学时），经中医药专业学术团体或医疗机构推荐者。

B.2.4 高级专科医师

参加高级专科医师测试的人员应至少符合以下要求中的 1 项：

（1）取得专科医师资格后，临床实践 5 年以上；或取得中医临床博士学位，中医临床实践 2 年以上；或取得中医临床硕士学位，中医临床实践 7 年以上。

（2）中医本科学历，从事临床医疗工作 11 年以上；或中医大专学历，从事临床医疗工作 14 年以上；或中医中专学历，从事临床医疗工作 16 年以上。

（3）取得其他非医学类本科学士学位，参加中医药学专业培训累计满 2500 学时（理论学习时间不少于 1500 学时），中医临床实践 11 年以上。

（4）家传、师承或自学中医，以中医为职业，从医 25 年以上；或从医 20 年以上，参加中医药培训累计满 3000 学时（理论学习时间不少于 2000 学时）。

B.2.5 主任医师

参加主任医师测试的人员应至少符合以下要求中的 1 项：

（1）取得高级专科医师资格后，临床实践 5 年以上；或取得中医临床博士学位，中医临床实践 7 年以上；或取得中医临床硕士学位，中医临床实践 12 年以上。

（2）中医本科学历，从事临床医疗工作 16 年以上；或中医大专学历，从事临床医疗工作 19 年以上；或中医中专学历，从事临床医疗工作 21 年以上。

（3）取得其他非医学类本科学士学位，参加中医药学专业培训累计满 2500 学时（理论学习时间不少于 1500 学时），中医临床实践 16 年以上。

（4）家传、师承或自学中医，以中医为职业，从医 30 年以上；或从医 25 年以上，参加中医药学专业培训累计满 3000 学时（理论学习时间不少于 2000 学时）。

附录 C

（资料性）
命题卡示例

考试科目：试题编号：（　　）

题　型	A₁	A₂	B₁	认知层次	记忆　理解　应用
试题在考试大纲中分布					细目
试题内容：					

标准答案		A.	B.	C.	D.	E.
标准答案出处						
主　题　词						
预计难度	命题专家判定	易　较易　中　较难　难				
	复审专家判定	易　较易　中　较难　难				
	审定专家判定	易　较易　中　较难　难				
命　题　人		命题时间				
复　审　人		复审日期				
审　定　人		审定日期				

附录 D

（资料性）

命题细目表示例

题号	大纲分布		认知层次			题型结构			预计难度					标准答案出处（教材版本与页码）	试题关键词
	单元	细目	理解	记忆	应用	A_1	A_2	B_1	难	较难	中	较易	易		

（表头"试题参数"横跨"大纲分布、认知层次、题型结构、预计难度"四项）

Foreword

Chief Drafting Organization: Committee of Examination and Evaluation of WFCMS, The Department of Examination and Accreditation of WFCMS, Beijing University of Chinese Medicine.

Chief Drafters: Zheng Yaoxian, Gao Sihua, Gao Wenzhu, Xu Jinxiang, Li Zhenji, Xu Chunbo, Zhai Shuangqing, Zhang Liping, Tang Mingke, Gu Xiaojing, Bao Wenhu.

Participating Drafters:

China: Jiang Zaizeng, Chen Lixin, Gu Xiaohong, Ding Xia, Wu Yufeng, Qing Shukun, Xiao Junping, Zhao Baixiao, Yan Xiaotian, Yang Shuning, Zhang Huazuo, Sun Qi, Yu Shuseng, Yu Wendi.

Singapore: Zhao Yingjie.

Brazil: Shi Hong, Ma Peiling.

Mexico: Song Qinfu, Li Meihong.

USA: Jin Ming.

Hungary: Yu Funian, Xia Linjun.

Canada: Wu Binjiang.

Japan: Chen Jianying.

Switzerland: Li Yiming.

Italy: He Jialang.

The standard is drafted in accordance with the rules given in the *SCM 0001-2009 Working Regulation for Formulation and Publication of Standard*.

The standard is reviewed and passed in the 6th session of the 3rd Board of World Federation of Chinese Medicine Societies held in Russia.

The Standard is issued by the World Federation of Chinese Medicine Societies. All rights reserved by the World Federation of Chinese Medicine Societies.

Introduction

To construct the standard system for talents of Chinese medicine is an important part of the international Chinese medicine talents strategy. *The Test and Assessment Procedures for Chinese Medicine Doctors*, which give the basic elements, indexes, content and methods to test and assess the acknowledge and clinical capability, will be helpful in promoting the quality of Chinese medicine talents.

Aiming to promote the test and assessment of international professional titles to step on the track of scientificalization and standardization, bases on the survey and research and according to the procedures of regulation for the international standard, the *Test and Assessment Procedures for International Chinese Medicine Doctors* been drafted.

The standard refers to the doctor management regulation of China, USA, Japan, UK and other countries or regions. It also refers to the relative standards of WFCMS. The standard gives relative requirements to guide and regulate the test and assessment for Chinese medicine doctors.

The standard is in line with the *SCM 0003 – 2009 World Standard of Chinese Medicine Undergraduate (Pre-CMD) Education* (includes its annex A) and *SCM 0010–2012 World Core Courses of Chinese Medicine Specialty*.

Apply to the *SCM 0008 – 2011 World Classification Standard for Professional Titles of Chinese Medicine Doctors*, the standard classifies the Chinese medicine doctors into assistant doctor, licensed doctor, specialist, senior specialist, and chief physician.

Written examinations and practical operations have been taking as main test methods, paper and medical case record review, thesis defense have been taking as main assessment methods in the standard.

The standard aims to give basic contents, methods and procedures for relative examination, assessment and evaluation of Chinese medicine doctors. It can be used in Chinese medicine doctors' ability examination and assessment, college examination or teacher assessment in countries or regions. Based on the standard, the countries or regions can set up their own management system about test and assessment for Chinese medicine doctors to ensure the safety and quality of service of Chinese medicine for the people all over the world.

Test and Assessment Procedures for International Chinese Medicine Doctors

1 Scope

This standard provides basic contents, methods and test and assessment procedures targeting on Chinese medicine (CM) doctors.

This standard is intent to be used in theoretical level and clinical technical skills certifications of CM doctors in different hierarchies and specialities no matter who have been or are going to be engaged in CM clinic.

2 Normative References

The following documents are indispensable when applying test and assessment standards. If documents are dated, only the dated versions are selected as quotations and references. If documents are not dated, the latest versions including all modifications are taken as references.

SCM 0003 *World Standard of Chinese Medicine Undergraduate (Pro-CMD) Education*

SCM 0008 *World Classification Standard for Professional Titles of Chinese Medicine Doctors*

SCM 0010 *World Core Courses of Chinese Medicine Speciality*

3 Terms and Definitions

3.1 Test

The process of theoretical level of CM and clinical skill test on examination candidate by written examination (to answer on the sheet by ball-point pen or pen), clinical technical operation, and syndrome differentiation and treatment in written form.

3.2 Assessment

The process of candidate's thesis reviewed by peers and proved medical records and thesis defense verified by peer experts in order to make judgment on the levels of CM theory, clinical and scientific research, and teaching.

3.3 Professional Training

The process of learning CM theory and clinical skill in different ways.

3.4 Clinical Practice

The process of being engaged in CM clinic by applying professional knowledge like Chinese herbal medicine, acupuncture and moxibustion, and tuina, etc. under the theory of CM.

3.5 Syndrome Differentiation and Treatment in Written Form

The process that examination candidate makes the diagnosis of disease and pattern, puts forward therapeutic method, and prescription including the selecting points in acupuncture and moxibustion and tuina as well as the corresponding operational approaches through the thought of syndrome differentiation in CM theory based on the provided medical case in written form.

4 Relative Responsibilities

4.1 Test and Assessment Institution

4.1.1 Institution carrying out the test and assessment for CM doctors shall be organizations such as Chinese medical hospitals, educational institutions, and CM association and so forth and these institution shall also meet the following basic conditions:

a) The related requirements regulated by the targeted country or local area;

b) Experts qualifying for question setting, test, and assessment as well as the execution of test personnel;

c) The place, equipment, and facilities required on test and assessment;

4.1.2 Establish the test and assessment committee made up of experts from different specialities in CM, and makes clear about their duties and working procedures. Drafting administrative rules shall cover the whole process of assessment in order to guarantee the quality of assessment.

4.2 Test and Assessment Organizer

Test and assessment organizer shall take responsibility of preliminary check on the qualification based on the application, recommendation, and execution of training for the qualified candidate.

4.3 Test and Assessment Implementer

Assessment implementer shall recheck the qualifications of these candidates and carry out assessment based on related rules.

4.4 Test and Assessment Applicants

4.4.1 The applicants of test and assessment of CM doctors shall be these people who have been engaged in or are going to be engaged in CM clinic by systematic learning.

4.4.2 Study and working experience in these applicants shall be qualified for the corresponding grade of CM test and assessment.

5 Test and Assessment Classification

5.1 Test

5.1.1 The test aims to check whether these candidates have possessed the basic knowledge and skills as a CM doctor or not.

5.1.2 The testing methods principally include written examination and clinical technical operation.

5.1.3 If the applicant passes these tests, the applicant can obtain the certificate for assistant doctors, licensed doctors or specialists.

5.2 Assessment

5.2.1 Comprehensive abilities and levels of professional theory, medical treatment, scientific research and teaching in these candidates shall be mainly examined.

5.2.2 The assessment modes include applicant's thesis reviewed by peers and proved medical records and thesis defense verified by peer experts.

5.2.3 If he or she passed the assessment, the CM doctor in clinical field can obtain the title of senior specialist or chief physician.

6 Methods

6.1 Written Examination

6.1.1 Range of Application and Form

6.1.1.1 Basic medical theory of CM, mastery of medical knowledge, and application ability of CM clinical knowledge shall be examined by written examination.

6.1.1.2 Choice question and question of syndrome differentiation and treatment in written form shall be tested by written examination.

6.1.2 Subjects in Written Examination

6.1.2.1 Major in CM

The related knowledge of basic theories of Chinese medicine, diagnostics of Chinese medicine, science of Chinese materia medica, formula study, internal medicine of Chinese medicine, surgery of Chinese medicine, gynecology of Chinese medicine, pediatrics of Chinese medicine, and syndrome differentiation and treatment in common diseases and frequently-occurring diseases are tested in written form.

6.1.2.1.1 Major in CM (for the Orientation of Acupuncture and Moxibustion)

The related knowledge of basic theory of Chinese medicine, human anatomy, study of meridians and acupuncture points, and clinical acupuncture, and syndrome differentiation and treatment in common diseases and frequently-occurring diseases are tested in written form.

6.1.2.1.2 Major in CM (for the Orientation of Tuina)

The related knowledge of basic theory of Chinese medicine, human anatomy, study of meridians and acupuncture points, and traditional Chinese tuina, and syndrome differentiation and treatment in common diseases and frequently-occurring diseases are tested in written form.

6.1.2.1.3 Major in CM (for the Orientation of Cosmetology)

Basic theory of Chinese medicine, science of Chinese materia medica and formula study, basic knowledge of CM cosmetology, clinical technique of CM cosmetology as well as syndrome differentiation and treatment on frequently-occurring diseases damaging beauty are tested in written form.

6.1.2.1.4 Major in CM (for the Orientation of Traumatology and Orthopedics)

Basic theory of Chinese medicine, human anatomy, study of meridians and acupuncture points, traditional Chinese tuina, traumatology and orthopedics of Chinese medicine are tested.

6.2 Clinical Technical Operation Examination

6.2.1 Clinical technical operation examination shall target on testing the basic clinical skills and the ability to solve the clinical practical disorders.

6.2.2 The operational abilities of clinical techniques including regular disinfection, location of acupoint, needling methods in common use of filiform needle, moxibustion technique, tuina, cupping, bone setting, sinew regulating, and plinlet fixing are mainly tested.

6.3 Assessment

6.3.1 CM doctor assessment shall take peer review as the major method.

6.3.2 The assessment shall focus on the basic theory of CM, clinical operation, scientific research, teaching, and mastery and application abilities of theories in CM classics.

6.4 Thesis Defense

6.4.1 The thesis defense refers to the comprehensive assessments on contestant's clinical thinking ability, scientific research quality, and literature quotation, etc. by answering expert's questions face to face based on peer-reviewed thesis.

6.4.2 The thesis defense shall assess the clinical critical thinking skills and scientific research quality in CM in the way of answering questions that targeted on the weak points, related academic arguments, new therapy, related diagnostic criteria, criteria of therapeutical effect, and relevant data involved in the thesis.

7 Working Process of Test

7.1 Determine Test Syllabuses

7.1.1 The implementer of test and assessment shall publish or post the test syllabus in an appropriate way for the convenience of obtaining by applicants before the test.

7.1.2 Specific scope of assessment shall be explicitly stipulated in test syllabus.

7.2 Formulate Test Implement Scheme

Contents of test item types, forms, total score, and minimum passing score shall be defined in the Test Implement Scheme.

7.3 Select Experts of Questions Setting

7.3.1 The experts of questions setting shall possess the stipulated educational background, and usually have technical titles of associate senior CM doctor or above.

7.3.2 The experts of questions setting shall be familiar with the theory and clinical skills, and know the development in relative fields.

7.3.3 The experts of questions setting shall be familiar with the technical rules of setting and analyzing questions.

7.4 Determine Question Setting Task

7.4.1 Question setting scheme shall be formulated to make clear relevant parameters such as the number of questions, test item types, cognitive level, and predicted difficulty.

7.4.2 Question setting scheme shall ensure the main knowledge points be reasonably covered in these tests.

7.5 Basic Rules in Questions Setting

7.5.1 Scope of questions setting shall follow the test syllabus.

7.5.2 The content of tests shall comprehensively cover main knowledge points of the test syllabus.

7.5.3 Tricky question, catch question, or question seldom occurred in clinic as well as controversial contents in academy should be avoided.

7.5.4 The content of tests shall be scientific and rigorous. Terms and nomenclatures shall be accurate and units of measurement shall be normalized.

7.5.5 One test item shall only give one single question.

7.5.6 Misapprehensive expressions on discriminations of race, religion, disability, and gender shall be avoided.

7.5.7 Figures involved in the test questions shall be unified in Arabic numerals.

7.5.8 Privative in question-stem shall be marked in boldface and overstriking.

7.5.9 The predicted difficulties in test questions shall comprise 5 levels: difficulty, relative difficulty, medium difficulty, relativeeasiness, and easiness.

7.6 Main Process and Requirements of Questions Setting

7.6.1 The experts of question setting shall work out question setting plan, and fill in detail table of question setting according to parameters specified in question setting scheme.

7.6.2 Question setting can be conducted after the accuracy of the detail table of question setting reasonably covers main knowledge points and logical relationship of each parameter to be sure.

7.6.3 Question setting card shall be filled standardly, and any item shall not be omitted.

7.6.4 The source of standard answers of question, including name, version, and page of the textbook, shall be labeled correctly.

7.6.5 Keywords of the question shall be extracted accurately.

7.6.6 The expert shall check the keywords of questions by himself/herself to ensure no reduplicative questions and reasonable distribution of questions.

7.6.7 Stetted questions can be submitted for rechecking after self-check that aims to ensure no wrong questions or wrong written characters in questions and to meet the parameters specified in question setting scheme.

7.7 Structure of Question Types

7.7.1 Choice Question

7.7.1.1 A_1 - Type Choice Question

Each test question shall be made up of one stem and 5 alternative answers. The stem shall be expressed in narrative simple sentence. Among 5 alternative answers, only one is the optimal choice for the question, which is named correct answer. The rest 4 answers shall all belong to distractors. The distractors can be completely wrong or partly correct.

7.7.1.2 A_2 - Type Choice Question

One simple medical case or two relevant factors or above shall be set as the question-stem, and 5 alternative answers related to the stem are following. Symptoms, tongue and tongue coating, and pulse condition shall all be listed. If disease condition is not related to gender or age, then these two basic information can be omitted. On answering the question, one out of 5 alternative choices shall be selected as correct answer.

7.7.1.3 B_1 - Type Choice Question

Test question shall be composed of several alternative answers and two question-stems or above. The alternative answers shall be listed before the stems. On answering the question, one out of 5 alternative choices can be selected as correct answer for each stem. Every alternative choices can be selected once or more, or none.

7.7.1.4 Question-stem Expression

The following rules shall be complied:

a) No punctuation in the end of question-stem;

b) Proportion of negative questions is not too high;

c) Double negation is inappropriate in question-stem;

d) For B_1 - type choice question, two stems share 5 alternative answers. The expression form of the two stems is consistent, and the contents belong to the same category.

7.7.1.5 Alternative Answer

The following basic principles shall be complied:

a) Contents of 5 alternative answers shall in the same category;

b) There shall not be any subsumption or hint among 5 alternative answers;

c) If they relate to figures, they shall be sequenced from the smallest to the largest, or from the largest to the smallest;

d) Distractor shall make the examinee feel confused or puzzled in a certain degree.

7.7.1.6 Correct Answer

The followingbasic principles shall be complied:

a) Based on the prescribed textbook or guide for test;

b) Accurately mark the version and specific page number of textbook or guide for correct answer.

7.7.2 Test-Question for Clinical Technical Operation

7.7.2.1 The basic skills related to the involved majors shall mainly be focused on.

7.7.2.2 The answer shall be correct, and standard for assessment shall be fair and rational.

7.7.3 Test-Question for Syndrome Differentiation and Treatment in Written Form

7.7.3.1 The following information shall be correctly provided:

a) Patient's name, gender, age, nationality, marital status, birthplace, occupation, solar terms of disease attack, and narrator of medical history;

b) Chief complaint: explicitly express patient's main symptoms or signs as well as time of duration, which cause patient to visit doctor;

c) History of present illness: According to clinical thinking of syndrome differentiation in CM, describe the main symptoms (signs), tongue appearance, pulse condition, and process of diagnosis and treatment since disease attack;

d) Past medical history: past health condition, disease history, and allergic history;

e) Personal history, marital and reproductive history, menstrual history, and family history related to syndrome differentiation.

7. 7. 3. 2   Test Contents in Item of Syndrome Differentiation and Treatment in Written Form

a) Diagnosis: both disease and syndrome in CM;

b) Therapeutic method: therapeutic method targeting on disease and syndrome diagnosis in CM, acupuncture and moxibustion, tuina, orthopaedics and traumatology, and cosmetology;

c) Prescription: the selected formula, main and adjunct acupuncture points, location for tuina, hand manipulation, bone setting, sinew regulating, and cosmetic technique;

d) Composition of prescription: Chinese herbs or acupoints are modified from a selected formula based on disease condition;

e) The dosages of all Chinese herbs, package, decocting method and instructions about how to take medicine are needed. The related expressions of hand manipulations are also necessary;

f) Doctor's advice: give some advice on nursing.

7. 8   Rules for Question-Review

7. 8. 1   In order to guarantee the quality of test questions, the procedures of self-check, recheck, and validation shall be carried out strictly.

7. 8. 2   Main contents for review should include:

a) Whether test contents go beyond the syllabus;

b) Whether structure of question types is correct;

c) Whether questions in the stem is clear understanding;

d) Whether alternative choices belong to the same category;

e) Recheck the source of correct answer;

f) Verify all distractors cannot be correct answers in optimal choices;

g) Whether extractions of subject terms in test questions are correct;

h) Whether there are wrongly written or mispronounced characters.

7. 9   Construction of Question Bank

7. 9. 1   Specially-assigned person responsible for the management of question warehouse shall be appointed.

7. 9. 2   Question warehouse shall be marked by course name for test, and each item has an only serial number.

7. 9. 3   The amount of test questions in question warehouse shall be determined by requirement.

7. 9. 4   The total test questions in each course shall not be less than 5 times compared with those selected in a test paper.

7. 9. 5   Test questions shall be updated and completed periodically based on changes of test syllabus and testing targets.

7. 9. 6   Security stipulations shall be strictly complied to ensure the security of question bank.

7. 10   Organizing Examination Paper

7. 10. 1   *The Plan of Organizing Examination Paper* shall be formulated in accordance with the level of

the examinee and the purpose of examination.

7. 10. 2   *The Plan of Organizing Examination Paper* shall clearly specify the requirement of every parameter of the ratio of the type of questions, expecting degree of difficulty, level of cognition, etc.

7. 10. 3   The examination question shall properly cover the main knowledge points.

7. 10. 4   In accordance with the stipulation of the examination, two papers of A and B shall be prepared for every examination in principle.

7. 10. 5   Make sure that Paper A and Paper B are equivalent with each other basically.

7. 11   Examination Paper Reviewing

7. 11. 1   After organizing the paper, in accordance with 7. 8 Stipulations of Reviewing Questions, at least two persons shall re-examine every test question of the paper. Any problem founded shall be submitted to the people of organizing examination paper for revising and perfecting.

7. 11. 2   The senior experts complete re-examining the paper.

7. 11. 3   The people responsible for formulating the questions of examination shall complete the examination paper reviewing.

7. 12   Warehousing the Examination Paper

7. 12. 1   Separately warehouse on the basis of the examination subjects.

7. 12. 2   Only one code for each paper.

7. 12. 3   Make registration on the basis of majors and time of organizing paper.

7. 13   Starting Using the Examination Paper

7. 13. 1   Going through the three-level procedure of reviewing paper.

7. 13. 2   Make accurate registration for the time of starting using and the applying country (region).

7. 14   Printing and Storing of the Paper

7. 14. 1   At least two persons together complete printing, separating and binding of the first paper.

7. 14. 2   Together verify the accuracy of the amount of questions, order of question numbers, page order, etc. in the paper.

7. 14. 3   The examination staff undertakes the responsibility of reading-through. After confirming that there is no mistake, complete printing the paper.

7. 14. 4   At least two persons re-verify the content on continuation of question order, integrity of questions in every page, page continuation, etc.

7. 14. 5   Verify the amount of the printed paper and seal for keeping in the confidential cabinet.

7. 15   Statistical Analysis

7. 15. 1   Make statistical analysis for differential validity of the examination question after examination.

7. 15. 2   Create conditions for marking the degree of difficulty of actual examination of the question.

7. 15. 3   If condition permits, conduct analysis for reliability and validity of the questions, as well as for the value of equivalence of the questions and examination papers.

7. 16   Examination Management

7. 16. 1   Sign-up of Examination

7. 16. 1. 1   In advance make public the information of sign-up and provide with related consultation of the examination.

7. 16. 1. 2   The candidate shall submit the sign-up form and related certificates at the appointed time.

7. 16. 1. 3   The implementation party of examination shall issue the examination permit after verifying the candidate's personnel information and qualification.

7. 16. 2 Staff of Examination

7. 16. 2. 1 Include one chief examiner and one monitor. If there exists a major of clinical technical operation in the examination, there must be at least one expert of the corresponding major.

7. 16. 2. 2 Arrange translators if needed.

7. 16. 3 Condition for the Chief Examiner

7. 16. 3. 1 Have the senior professional title of Chinese Medicine, and be familiar with administrative rules of examination.

7. 16. 3. 2 Perform one's duty honestly and exercise strict self-discipline, conduct examination impartially, and abide by the discipline of privacy consciously.

7. 16. 3. 3 Have the stronger ability to manage and coordinate examination.

7. 16. 4 Responsibility of the Chief Examiner

7. 16. 4. 1 Be responsible for implementation of examination according to related regulations of examination.

7. 16. 4. 2 Properly deal with the emergency occurred during the examination.

7. 16. 5 Condition of Monitor

7. 16. 5. 1 Have the intermediate or above technical professional title of Chinese medicine.

7. 16. 5. 2 Perform one's duty honestly and exercise strict self-discipline, conduct examination impartially, and abide by the discipline of privacy consciously.

7. 16. 6 Responsibility of Monitor

7. 16. 6. 1 Coordinate with the chief examiner to do well in related management work in the examination place.

7. 16. 6. 2 Complete every task of work assigned by the chief examiner.

7. 16. 6. 3 Be responsible for matters of recycling and sealing of the answer sheet, arranging practice of examination, etc.

7. 16. 7 Condition of Translator

7. 16. 7. 1 Be proficient in the language of the examination, and have the work experience of professional translation for at least three years.

7. 16. 7. 2 Be familiar with the knowledge of Chinese medicine.

7. 16. 8 Responsibility of Translator

7. 16. 8. 1 Undertake the task of translation at the examination place, and accurately translate the content of questions and answers which shall not disobey the original idea.

7. 16. 8. 2 Abide by administrative rules of the examination, and it is not allowed to cue the examinee without authorization.

7. 16. 9 Regulations of the Examination

7. 16. 9. 1 The institution of examination shall formulate regulation of the examination room, so as to regulate the behavior of the examinee and make clear the related measures of punishment.

7. 16. 9. 2 The institution of examination shall formulate regulations of the examination, so as to regulate the behavior of the examiner and guarantee the impartialness and justice of the examination.

7. 16. 10 Deployment of the Examination

7. 16. 10. 1 The examination place shall be located in the area with easy access and quiet environment.

7. 16. 10. 2 The schedule of examination shall be posted at the remarkable place of examination.

7. 16. 10. 3 Separate row and separate desk for an examinee, and the interval all round shall be no less

than 80 cm.

7.16.10.4 Post the number of examinee on the upper left corner of the desk in order.

7.16.11 Preparation of the Examination

7.16.11.1 The staff of the examination shall verify the information of examination paper and related appliance of examination according to the schedule of examination one by one.

7.16.11.2 The staff of examination shall check the examination place in detail according to the requirement of layout of the examination place.

7.16.12 Procedure of Examination

7.16.12.1 Written Examination

7.16.12.1.1 Before start of examination the chief examiner introduce the members of the examination group, rules of examination room, related information of examination and matters needing attention.

7.16.12.1.2 Unsealing the examination sheet: the staff of examination shall not unseal the envelop of examination paper until show the examinee that the sealing of the examination sheet is in good condition.

7.16.12.1.3 Distributing examination paper: the examination paper, answer sheet and rough paper shall be distributed by the staff of examiner, but not passed by examinee.

7.16.12.1.4 After the chief examiner announces the beginning of examination, the examinee starts.

7.16.12.1.5 Verifying information: The monitor shall check the information of examinee, photo of the examination permit, photo of valid certificate. If there exist questions, report to the chief examiner timely.

7.16.12.1.6 Cue of ending: twenty minutes before the ending of examination, the staff of examiner shall cue the examinee the time.

7.16.12.1.7 Ending of examination: after making the signal of examination, the examinee shall stop answering, and put the examination paper and answer sheet on the desk and then exit the examination room.

7.16.12.1.8 Sealing examination paper: the staff of examination shall collect and put in order the answer sheet according to the order of numbers, and put the record of examination in the special envelope of answer sheet for sealing.

7.16.12.1.9 At least two persons shall sign names and time.

7.16.12.2 Clinical Practice

7.16.12.2.1 Select questions to prepare examination: the examinee shall be in the waiting area to randomly draw off the questions five minutes in advance.

7.16.12.2.2 Technical practice: the examinee shall enter into the examination room one by one, and state and display the content of practice.

7.16.12.2.3 Scoring: at least two staffs of examination scores respectively according to the standard answer and calculate the average value as the score of the examinee.

7.16.12.2.4 Sealing examination paper: after examination, the staff of examination shall put the transcripts and examination paper into the envelope and then make signature.

7.16.13 Report of Examination

It shall cover the following content:

a) Major of examination, batch of the examination, amount of examinees (first examination, make-up examination), country of examination, city of examination, organizer of examination (group or individual).

b) Qualification of examinee: nationality, academic background, profession, age, etc.

c) The previous situation of organizing examination of this examination place: major of examination, level, batch of examination, amount of examination in every year; amount and time for assessment of senior professional title.

d) The existing main problems: be mainly related to management of examination, qualification of questions of examination paper, etc. ; main advice and suggestion of the organizer of the examination.

e) Related situation of expanding of examination.

f) Thought and suggestion of the group of examiners.

7. 17　Scoring Examination Paper

7. 17. 1　The staff of examination and person of scoring paper shall fulfill The List Delivery and Receipt of Examination Paper and Answer Sheet.

7. 17. 2　The person of scoring paper shall have technical professional title on Chinese medicine.

7. 17. 3　They shall score at the assigned place together, and the examination paper and answer sheet are forbidden to take out of the place of scoring paper.

7. 17. 4　Based on the standard answer offered by the department of management of examination paper, score the paper with red pen.

7. 17. 5　A same examination paper shall be scored by at least two persons. Make a signature at the assigned place after completion of scoring.

7. 17. 6　The person of verifying examination shall conscientiously verify the scores. If error of scoring occurs, correct it and then make a signature. If there exists a dispute, it shall be judged by the department of examination.

7. 17. 7　Complete scoring and statistics of scores three weeks after examination in principle.

7. 17. 8　After recording scores, no one can correct the scores of examinee without authorization.

7. 18　Management of Archives

7. 18. 1　Archives management regulations shall be set up.

7. 18. 2　Related data of the information of examinee, answer sheet, transcripts, etc. shall be kept in file according to archives management regulations.

8　Working Process of Assessment

8. 1　Procedure of Application

8. 1. 1　The institution of assessment shall make clear the requirement of qualification of academic background, number of years of employment, etc.

8. 1. 2　The applicant shall fulfill the application form factually and make relative declaration about whether is there any law-breaching records during practicing.

8. 1. 3　The organizer of assessment shall assesse the data of applicants according to the requirement of qualification made by the institution of assessment on the academic background, number of years of employment, etc.

8. 1. 4　For the applicant who meets the qualification, his or her working unit (the cooperation, hospital, university, etc.) or two persons who have the senior professional title of Chinese Medicine shall issue recommendation letter.

8. 2　Submit the Documents of Assessment

8. 2. 1　Publish two academic paper of Chinese medicine, and the number of words of every paper shall be no less than 3000.

8. 2. 2　There shall be at least 10 valid cases covering five or more different diseases.

8. 2. 3　If the applicant uses other minority languages except English to write paper, the abstracts in Chinese and English are both needed.

8.3 Verification of Qualification

The institution of assessment shall verify the application documents and confirm whether the applicant has the qualification of participating in assessment of qualification.

8.4 Assessment of the Peer Review

8.4.1 According to the content of paper and case, select two or more experts of the same occupation for assessment.

8.4.2 The experts of assessment in principle shall have the professional title of chief physician, professors or researcher.

8.4.3 The paper and case shall be submitted two months before oral defense of the paper.

8.4.4 Main contents of assessment in the paper should include:

a) Continuity of thought on clinical practice of Chinese medicine;

b) Correctness of application of theory of Chinese medicine;

c) Scientific character of clinical research of Chinese medicine;

d) Accuracy of literature review;

e) Truthfulness of related documents;

f) Validity of clinical treatment;

g) Innovation of clinical research;

h) Logicality of related analysis;

i) Exactness of conclusion of paper;

j) Usefulness of guiding clinical practice.

8.4.5 Main contents of assessment of the case should include:

a) Truthfulness of case; logicality and accuracy of description of case;

b) Accuracy of syndrome of Chinese medicine, and diagnosis for type of syndrome;

c) Rationality of treatment, prescription and medicine (main acu-point, matching acu-points, tuina, bone-setting);

d) Reliability of courses of treatment;

e) Other questions related to the case.

8.4.6 Opinions of assessment

8.4.6.1 The institution of assessment shall give the following opinion of assessment according to the situation of assessment from the same occupation:

a) Reach the same level and agree to participate in oral defense of paper;

b) When being advised to perfect the paper and case, temperately disagree to participate in oral defense of paper.

8.4.6.2 The institution of assessment shall timely give feedback on conclusion of assessment to the applicants.

8.5 Implementing Oral Defense of Paper

8.5.1 The committee of oral defense shall be made up of 5 ~ 7 experts with the professional title of related majors of chief physician (pharmaceutist), professors or researcher.

8.5.2 The applicant shall report the abstract of paper for 15 minutes, and the time for experts' questions and for oral defense shall be 25 minutes in total.

8.5.3 If other languages except Chinese are needed for oral defense, 10 ~ 15 minutes for oral defense can be added properly and the translator shall promise to translate accurately.

8. 5. 4 The experts of the committee of oral defense shall separately score.

8. 5. 5 After making statistics of scores, the committee of oral defense shall discuss and make the following conclusion:

a) pass the oral defense;

b) the paper is needed to be re-assessed after rectification;

c) not pass the oral defense.

8. 5. 6 Submit to the assessment committee of technical professional title of Chinese medicine for verification.

8. 6 Result of Assessment

8. 6. 1 The result of examination and assessment shall be submitted to the committee of assessment for verification.

8. 6. 2 Timely and accurately make public the result of assessment.

9 Management of Certificate

9. 1 Formulate the certificate for applicants who passed the examination and assessment according to the result of committee of examination and assessment.

9. 2 Complete notification of certification in two months.

9. 3 If there exists a situation of false qualification, juvenile record, etc. of the applicant, the institution of assessment shall revoke the issued certificate of assessment and report to the organizer of examination.

Annex A

(Informative)
Sample of Question Type

A. 1　Multiple-Choice of Written Examination

A. 1. 1　Sample of Question Type A_1

Whose characteristic of the following pathogenic qi is heavy and turbid (explanatory form)?

A. wind

B. summer-heat qi

C. dampness

D. dryness

E. cold

Answer: C

A. 1. 2　Sample of Question Type A_2

A. 1. 2. 1　Sample 1

The patient feels forgetful and sleepless, vertiginous and ear-ringing, hot hands, feet and heart, painful side of body and waist, dry mouth and throat, red tongue and little saliva, small and weak pulse. The syndrome is

A. deficiency of kidney yin

B. deficiency of heart yin

C. deficiency of liver and kidney yin

D. deficiency of the liver blood

E. deficiency of lung and kidney yin

Answer: C

A. 1. 2. 2　Sample 2

Patient, female, 28 years old, married. After gestation she feels that the costal and hypochondiac region are swelling and painful, she is impetuous and easy to be angry, the cover of tongue is thin and yellow, pulse is slippery. The formulas of first choice for treatment is

A. Peripatetic Powder

B. Minor Bupleurum Decoction

C. Major Bupleurum Decoction

D. Ass-hide glue and argyi leaf decoction

E. Angelica and Peony Powder

Answer: A

A. 1. 3　Sample of Question Type B_1

A. liver

B. heart

C. spleen

D. lung

E. kidney

The organ which nourishes the tendon and bone, so as to make body bear fatigue is Answer: A

The organ which has the closest relationship with nutrition situation of four limbs is Answer: C

A. 2 Sample of Question of syndrome differentiation and treatment in written form

Name of Patient	××	Gender	Male	Age	6	Status of Marriage	Single	Occupation	Banker
Address	Xicheng District, Beijing, China						Time of first Treatment		January 3rd, 2007

Interrogation:

Main complaint: fever with aversion to cold for one day.

Present medical history: he did not feel well from yesterday afternoon, was afraid of cold and had a fever, and became serious gradually. At present, he got a fever with aversion to cold, the syndrome of aversion to cold is serious while fever is comparatively mild, without sweat, with a headache, stuffy nose, thin nasal discharge sometimes, sneezing frequently, itching throat as well as thin white phlegm.

Previous medical history: healthy.

Inspection: thin but moistening cover of tongue.

Auscultation and olfaction: heavy and deep vocal sound.

Pulse-feeling and palpation: floating and tight pulse.

Answer for Reference

Diagnosis: diagnosing of name: influenza.

Diagnosing of type of syndrome: wind cold (exterior tightened by wind-cold).

Treatment: relieving the exterior with the warm pungent, freeing lung for dispelling cold.

Prescription: addition and subtraction of Antiphlogistic Powder of Schizonepetae and Ledebouriellae

Fineleaf Schizonepeta Herb 6g Divaricate Saposhnikovia Root 6g Incised Notopterygium Rhizome and Root 6g Doubleteeth Pubescent Angelica Root 6g Chinese Thorowax Root 6g Sichuan Lovage Rhizome 6g Hogfennel Root 6g Indian Bread 6g Orange Fruit 6g Platycodon Root 6g Liquorice Root 6g

Three dosages. One dosage per day, decoct with water and remove dregs to get juice, take it in the morning and evening separately.

Doctor's advice: preventing from wind and coldness, having rest, light meals, and avoiding the omophagia, cold, fried and the greasy food.

Signature of the doctor: ×××

Time of prescription: January 3rd, 2007

A. 3 Sample of Question of clinical practice

A. 3. 1 Example 1

Please confirm the detailed location of ST4 in the body, and briefly introduce the basis or key points of acupoint-selection.

Answer: in the face, outside the angle of mouth, upside straight to pupil.

A. 3. 2　Example 2

Inserting the needle by holding it.

Answer: Inserting the needle by pinch needle method, that is, using thumb and forefinger of left hand to hold the sterilized dry cotton ball, clamp the bottom of needle, fix the tip of needle at the surface of acu-point to be needled, twiddle the handle of needle with right hand, and needle it into the acu-point. The method applies needling for long needles.

Annex B

(Informative)

Classification and Application Requirements for International Chinese Medicine Doctors

B. 1 Classification

The professional technical titles of International Chinese Medicine Doctors can be classified into the following five levels:

1) assistant doctor

2) practicing doctor

3) specialist

4) senior specialist

5) chief physician

B. 2 Application Requirements

B. 2. 1 Assistant Doctor

The person who is to take part in examination of assistant doctor shall at least meet one of the following requirements:

1) After obtaining the professional title of intern doctor of Chinese medicine, more than three years of clinical practice.

2) For person with the academic background in Chinese medicine of a secondary technical school (three-year school system), more than three years of Chinese medicine clinical practice.

3) For person with the academic background in Chinese medicine of a junior college (three-year school system), at least one year of Chinese medicine clinical practice.

4) Taking part in CM professional training to accumulate for more than 1500 credit hours, and more than one year of Chinese medicine clinical practice.

5) For person learning Chinese medicine from family heritage, master-guiding-apprentice or self-study, being engaged in clinical work of Chinese medicine for more than five years, and being recommended by academic group or medical institution of Chinese medicine.

B. 2. 2 Practicing Doctor

The person who is to take part in examination of practicing doctor shall at least meet one of the following requirements:

1) After obtaining the professional tile of assistant doctor of Chinese medicine, more than three years of clinical practice.

2) Obtaining master's degree of Chinese medicine.

3) With an undergraduate academic background of Chinese medicine, more than one year of clinical practice.

4) With an academic background of junior college majoring in Chinese medicine, more than three years of clinical practice.

5) With an academic background of secondary school majoring in Chinese medicine, more than five years of clinical practice.

6) With a non-medical undergraduate or above academic background of Chinese medicine, taking part in CM professional training course to accumulate for more than 2500 credit hours (among which the time for theoretical study shall be more than 1500 credit hours), and more than one year of clinical practice.

7) For person learning Chinese medicine from family heritage, master-guiding-apprentice or self-study, being engaged in clinical practice of Chinese medicine for 12 years or above, and recommended by academic group and medical institution of Chinese medicine.

B. 2. 3　Specialist

The person who is to take part in the examination of specialist shall at least meet one of the following requirements:

1) After obtaining the professional title of practicing doctor of Chinese medicine, more than five years of clinical practice.

2) Obtaining doctor's degree of Chinese medicine.

3) After obtaining master's degree of Chinese medicine, more than two years of clinical practice.

4) With an undergraduate academic background of Chinese medicine, more than six years of clinical practice.

5) With an academic background of junior college majoring in Chinese medicine, more than nine years of clinical practice.

6) With an academic background of secondary school majoring in Chinese medicine, more than 11 years of clinical practice.

7) With an non-medical undergraduate or above background, taking part in training of Chinese medicine to accumulate for 2500 credit hours (the time for theoretical study shall be no less than 1500 credit hours), more than six years of clinical practice.

8) For person learning Chinese medicine from family heritage, master-guiding-apprentice or self-study, being engaged in clinical practice of Chinese medicine for 17 years or above, taking part in CM professional training to accumulate for 3000 credit hours (the time for theoretical study shall be no less than 2000 credit hours), and being recommended by academic group and medical institution of Chinese medicine.

B. 2. 4　Senior Specialist

The person who is to take part in the examination of senior specialist shall at least meet one of the following requirements:

1) After obtaining the qualification of specialist, more than five years of clinical practice; or obtain doctor's degree in clinical specialty of Chinese medicine, more than two years of clinical practice; or obtaining master's degree in in clinical specialty of Chinese medicine, more than seven years of clinical practice

2) With an undergraduate background in Chinese medicine, being engaged in clinical practice for more than 11 years; or with an academic background of junior college majoring in Chinese medicine, being engaged in the work of clinical practice for more than 14 years; or with an academic background of secondary school majoring in Chinese medicine, being engaged in clinical practice for more than 16 years.

3) Obtaining non-medical bachelor's degree, taking part in CM professional training to accumulate for 2500 credit hours (the time for theoretical study shall be no less than 1500 credit hours), more than 11 years of clinical practice of Chinese medicine.

4) For person learning Chinese medicine from family heritage, master-guiding-apprentice or self-study, being engaged in clinical practice of Chinese medicine for 25 years or above; or being engaged in clinical practice of Chinese medicine for 20 years or above, and taking part in training of Chinese medicine to

accumulate for 3000 credit hours (the time for theoretical study shall be no less than 2000 credit hours) .

B. 2. 5　Chief Physician

The person who is to take part in the examination of chief physician shall at least meet one of the following requirements:

1) After obtaining the qualification of senior specialist, be engaged in clinical practice for more than five years; or obtaining doctor's degree in clinical specialty of Chinese medicine, more than seven years of clinical practice of Chinese medicine; or obtaining master's degree in clinical practice of Chinese medicine, being engaged in clinical practice of Chinese medicine for more than 12 years.

2) With an undergraduate background, being engaged in clinical practice for more than 16 years; or with an academic background of junior college majoring in Chinese medicine, being engaged in clinical practice for 19 years or above; or with an academic background of secondary school, being engaged in clinical practice for more than 21 years.

3) Obtaining non-medical bachelor's degree, taking part in CM professional training to accumulate for 2500 credit hours (the time for theoretical study shall be no less than 1500 credit hours), and more than 16 years of clinical practice of Chinese medicine.

4) For person learning Chinese medicine from family heritage, master-guiding-apprentice or self-study, being engaged in clinical practice of Chinese medicine for 30 years or above; or being engaged in clinical practice of Chinese medicine for 25 years or above, and taking part in training of Chinese medicine to accumulate for 3000 credit hours (the time for theoretical study shall be no less than 2000 credit hours).

Annex C

(Informative)
Sample of Question Setting Sheet

Subject of Examination: Question No. : (   )

Type of Questions	A$_1$ ☐ A$_2$ ☐ B$_1$ ☐	Level of Cognition	Memory ☐ Comprehension ☐ Application ☐		
Distribution of Questions in the Outline of Examination			Detailed Items		
Content of Questions:					
Standard Answer		A. B. C. D. E.			
Reference for Standard Answer					
Keywords					
Expecting Degree of Difficulty	Grading by Expert of Formulating Questions	Easy ☐ Relative Easy ☐ Medium ☐ Relative Difficult ☐ Difficult ☐			
	Grading by Expert of Reviewing Questions	Easy ☐ Relative Easy ☐ Medium ☐ Relative Difficult ☐ Difficult ☐			
	Grading by Expert of Verifying Questions	Easy ☐ Relative Easy ☐ Medium ☐ Relative Difficult ☐ Difficult ☐			
Person of Formulating Questions		Time of Formulating Questions			
Person of Reviewing Questions		Date of Reviewing Questions			
Person of Verifying Questions		Date of Verifying Questions			

Annex D

(Informative)

Classification and Statistics Form for Question Setting

Question No.	Question Parameter														
	Distribution of the Outline		Level of Cognition			Structure of Question Type			Expecting Degree of Difficulty					Reference for Standard Answer (Edition and Page of the Textbook)	Key Words for Question
	Unit	Detailed Item	Compre-hension	Memory	Applica-tion	A_1	A_2	B_1	Difficulty	Relative Difficulty	Medium	Relative Easiness	Easiness		